MW01519303

Top 10 Excuses For Avoiding Exercise And How To Overcome Them

A Guide to Get You Started on the Right Path

Reggie Lamptey

authorHOUSE®

AuthorHouse™
1663 Liberty Drive
Bloomington, IN 47403
www.authorhouse.com
Phone: 1-800-839-8640

First published by AuthorHouse   6/17/2011

ISBN: 978-1-4634-2302-5 (sc)
ISBN: 978-1-4634-2304-9 (e)

Library of Congress Control Number: 2011910006

Printed in the United States of America

Any people depicted in stock imagery provided by Thinkstock are models, and such images are being used for illustrative purposes only. Certain stock imagery © Thinkstock.

This book is printed on acid-free paper.

Content Edited by ShaVaughn Morris & Glen Adamafio

TABLE OF CONTENTS

DEDICATION

This book is for all of those who struggle to find a way to reach your goals and dreams.
To all who always believed in me. Making sure to push me and never give up towards reaching my goals. I Love You!
If you believe, you can achieve.
Love yourself first and foremost.
Stay fit and healthy.

INTRODUCTION

You are not alone! You are not the only one who faces the many challenges that prevent people from being healthy; those issues that arise when it comes time to exercise because you feel obligated and not necessarily empowered. The intent of this book is just that, to empower and motivate you to achieve your goals and live a better, healthier lifestyle.

Let me ask you a few quick questions: 1. Do you think you'd be more health conscience if only your life wasn't so hectic or if your schedule wasn't so busy? 2. Do you find yourself getting comfortable at home and not wanting to get up and do some exercise? 3. Have you ever decided to start working out then given up because you felt you didn't know exactly what to do? My thought is that you've answered yes to either one or all of these questions. The good thing about your answer is that all of these issues and more, will be addressed and hopefully you'll be ready to move past them by the time you're finished reading.

Again, *you are not alone.* We all face the same issues. The difference between those of us who aren't reaching our goals and those of us who are; is not particularly because they have more free time or because it's required of their profession, they achieve it because they choose to set priorities and make things happen. It may be a tough thing to accept but there's only one viable reason why you don't meet your goals...you choose not to [insert shrug]. In most cases – I've found – people are not ready to make the adjustment, or lifestyle change that will enable them get to the next level. That's really the bottom line. People attempt to justify why they're not working out, beginning an exercise routine, or finding ways to eat healthier by calling them "reasons", in the end they are all just ***excuses***.

There are all types of excuses out there – some even seemingly justifiable – but they all can be conquered. At times people convert these excuses into "justifiable reasons", to make them feel OK about not getting started. I've seen people who desire to have a flashy car, live a glamorous lifestyle and keep up with the latest fashions. The funny thing is; these same people would never think to divert at least some of that time, energy, and money towards their own health. Since when did your health become last on the list of priorities? Yes, it's nice to have and want all these other things, but at what price are you willing to get them? Is it worth risking your own health for family or friends to praise you? Maybe these people should consider the old saying "your health is your wealth" because without good health, it would be hard to enjoy your wealth or even obtain it.

Through many conversations and interviews with different types of people, I've realized that the major cause of failure to attain goals is fear. Fear is almost always linked to an individual's excuse in one way or another. It could be a fear of not achieving your goal. Maybe you truly believe that your job has to be the number one priority in your life. OK here's what you probably haven't considered; if you neglect your health for too long you may end up with an issue that will keep you out of work, AND, if you don't go to work you may lose your job…but this is what you were trying to avoid by putting your employment first…wasn't it? So are you really making the right choice? Think about it hard.

It constantly amazes me how people so easily put their health on hold, or how they just can't seem to make living an overall healthier life part of their priorities. Why is decreasing the risk of serious health issues such as heart attack or diabetes, not important enough for people to make time to exercise or eat healthier food? What would you do if you went to the doctor and were told that you only have a few months left to live due to lack of health maintenance? What if he said "if you don't make some immediate changes, which include regular exercise and better eating habits, your time will be limited to a few months?" What would you do at that point? I'm sure that most people would begin to see their "reasons" as nothing more than excuses. They'd begin to make the changes necessary to prevent the unwanted outcome. BUT, is it really necessary to be within inches of the worst possible outcome before deciding to make change? The reality is; you will never overcome your excuses if you don't put the importance of your health into perspective. If you never give it thought then you will never see its importance. The sooner you realize that your health is your most important asset, the better off you will be.

Another point I want to make is that, you are not destined to look how your mother, father, or even grandparents looked. If you come from a family who's had poor eating or health habits for generations - it's OK. Remember, you can always be the one to break the tradition and begin a new one. We all have choices in life. You can make better choices than they did to avoid some of their issues. Making the choice not to have the same unhealthy eating habits is a start. Don't! I repeat, don't - beat yourself down by thinking that you're destined to end up the same way those in your family before you did. You can do better! You have the opportunity of taking advantage of the knowledge they chose not to, and you can make the choice to so.

Obviously, you can't change your height or your bone structure. Those things were passed down to you, but you can change your muscle tone and total body fat level, as well as the overall condition of your health. If you find yourself lacking the patience, focus, drive, or motivation needed to achieve your goal; remember that these traits were not passed down to you. Instead, they are things you develop. Since you are the one who develops these attributes, you have the power to change them.

Optimizing your health and wellness will give you many benefits. Benefits which are not limited to just looking good, they will also make you feel good and perform better. People tend to look at exercise just as a way of altering their physical appearance. They don't always consider the holistic or overall health benefits – those things that you can't see or don't seem immediately tangible. Starting simple and making gradual changes could have a great effect on your health and your life. With consistent exercise, you will begin to notice changes in the way your clothing fits, your energy levels, and even your work output.

In this book, I will give you strategies for understanding your excuses and ways to overcome them. Some of the strategies will include: 1) writing down your excuse(s), 2) brainstorming and explain the reasons for your excuse(s), 3) identifying real cause of the excuse(s), 4) creating and planning the steps to overcoming your excuse(s), and many more. Each chapter will outline one of the top 10 excuses and give you input on why you shouldn't let that excuse hold you back. It will also give you tips on how to move past the barrier and getting started. In order to help you better understand that you're not alone, I have interviewed 20 people of differing backgrounds and professions. Each person will give you their own personal reasons for working out and also explain how they've overcome their specific excuse. Not only will you have my input but you will have the input from these men and women to help you relate and feel connected. Hopefully, this will spark your decision to make a change and not let these excuses hold you back any longer.

"If you push yourself beyond your perceived limits nothing will ever be unattainable."

10 I'M TOO TIRED, AND I DON'T HAVE THE ENERGY TO...

Finishing the list at number 10 is the age-old, "I'm too tired" excuse. Many people who have busy and active lifestyles still find time to exercise! However, there are some minor differences which may separate you from them. Could it be that they chose to do something to change their consistent tiredness and lack of energy? Without giving it much thought, could you think of reasons that you may always be tired? Could you find the cause of you not having the energy to get through the day? If you knew the causes, would do something about it? There are ways to create more energy for yourself so you'll be less tired throughout the day.

One of the first steps is beginning a regular exercise program. This is the easiest and best way to increase your energy throughout the day. Once you begin you'll find yourself tired right after a workout, but as time passes, you'll see your energy increase; making you better equipped to handle the activities of the day. This is only one of the many benefits that you receive from regular exercise. If you continue your regimen, your desire to workout will outweigh your thoughts of feeling tired, and eventually the feeling of tiredness will start to fade away.

Second, changing your eating habits can help increase your overall level of energy. Lack of energy can usually be directed back to a person's eating habits. By making small changes to your eating habits, you can produce more energy and achieve an overall sense of well-being. Eliminating foods that are processed, high in fat or full of empty calories can help you from developing toxins in your body. These toxins pollute the body and strip it of essential nutrients that it needs to function optimally. Am I saying that you have to give up everything that's considered "junk food", no; however, reducing your consumption of it will reap great benefits to your health. Also, including natural foods in your diet will also deem beneficial to you. Eating fruits such as blueberries and oranges can help improve energy levels, as well as get much needed antioxidants into your body. Green vegetables like spinach are energy boosters as well. Look at Popeye what did he do when he needed strength and energy, he ate some spinach. Additionally, you should consider snacking on foods such as almonds, yogurt, or even dried fruits.

Many people stop when they begin to get tired. Oftentimes they stop because they are mentally weak and don't have the inner strength to push past the pain and tiredness. Pain is temporary, but the pride earned by achieving your goals lasts a lifetime. Why not push harder, if the results will benefit you for your lifetime? Other people will go until they are about to collapse. These people have the determination to succeed and would like to see achieve what they've set out to do come to fruition. The elite – the few who set out to become the very best – have the knowledge that their mind will grow weary and become weak before their body. With this knowledge, they continue to push themselves until all of their limits are shattered. By finding your motivation you can become one of the people who go beyond their limits.

Finding what works best for you will help you find the balance to succeed. This balance will keep you motivated, and will enable you to create more reasons to work towards your goals. There is a saying that a woman's work is never done. Lakisha Grant, Engineer and Real Estate agent is the Managing Director of the Audio and Visual Department of New Jersey City University. This woman stays busy and is involved in a number of different things, but somehow she always finds the energy to make sure she gets in a solid workout. In her spare time, she even plays in the Independent Woman's Football League (IWFL).

The level of importance and reasons for a person to want to workout can range and vary from person to person. Lakisha describes her need for working out below...

> *"Working out is important because I love being active, it helps me maintain the lifestyle I desire, it relieves stress, and boosts self-confidence. Working out is also important to me because as I age, my body will not breakdown as quickly as someone who leads a sedentary lifestyle. Exercising also helps you to look your best."*

More importantly, she enjoys exercise. She has found a way to make it more enjoyable which allows her to stay focused and continue doing it.

> *"I work out to stay in shape and to play sports. Working out helps me stay in optimum shape to have my body perform on the football field, reduce injuries, and be a top performer."*

With the large workload she has, working out enables her to reduce the stressors of everyday life. She is able to remain calm and focused.

At any point in her day Lakisha could find a reason to complain about being tired and not having the energy to do what she needs; yet, she doesn't! Her desire to achieve, and be the best, will not allow her to fall victim to this excuse. Of course there are times where she doesn't feel like doing anything more than she has to, but she always pushes herself to go that extra step.

> *"This excuse doesn't hold me back because once you start to exercise; you actually increase your energy levels."*

She can use that extra energy to power her through the day, in addition to helping her relax in the evening. If she didn't workout she wouldn't be able to perform the way she wants on the field.

> *"I know that I want to be able to still play on the team and have a starting position. Without continuous exercise I would fall behind and most likely lose my spot to someone who is pushing themselves harder than I am. Not starting is not an option for me. My goals in life as well as my desire to live a long healthy life will always keep me doing some form of exercise."*

The most important thing you can do is to take care of yourself.

Lakisha provides us with three tips for anyone who may find themselves saying they don't have the energy to workout.

"You can hire a personal trainer to help keep you motivated even though you may feel tired. You can also work out during the time of the day where you feel like your energy level is at its highest. Lastly just stop making excuses for not taking care of the number one person which is YOU!!!"

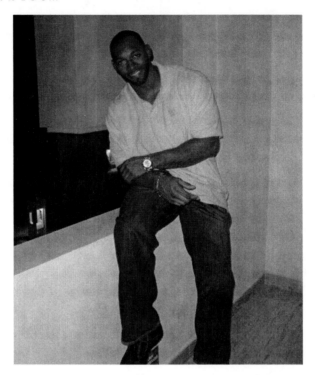

It's all about choices. You have the power to make the choice that will keep you focused and motivated. Darrin Davis, machine operator at Colgate Palmolive, full time student and part time personal trainer. He could easily fall victim to the "I'm too tired" excuse because he lives a life of constant activity, but he manages to stay focused and committed to find ways to still workout.

Darrin was also a former Division one football player at Southern Connecticut State. He played professionally in the AFL and XFL. He has carried on his athletic nature and drive, even though he has retired. As I've already said, everyone has their own reasons to workout. Some because they know the health benefits, others choose to because of vanity reasons.

Darrin simply does it because he just can't picture himself not being in shape

"I workout because it keeps me healthy and strong. I also workout because I love the way I look and feel when I do and I just simply love being in shape. I just couldn't sit and picture myself being a fat boy and unhealthy. Even though my career as a professional athlete is over, I've always been a competitive person by nature. Only now what I compete for is keeping myself healthy strong and staying alive as long as I can."

Despite being in the health and wellness field, he knows he would still workout no matter what.

"I am an athlete first and a personal trainer second. Working out is part of who I am, it's been embedded in my DNA. I wouldn't have it any other way. If I told myself that I was too tired and I didn't have the energy to do it, I would never get anything done. Not just working out, but a lot of things in my life wouldn't get done, because who doesn't get tired at some point?"

He sets his priorities so that his needs get taken care of before his wants. He works to get it all done. Even with everything that he has on his plate, he still finds the energy to workout. There are days where after a full day of school, he goes to work until 7am. Right after getting off, he would stop for some breakfast; go to the gym and workout. Now that is dedication!

"It doesn't take that much time for you to get in a good work out. You can start with as little as 20 to 30 minutes, or go more intense and do 60 to 90minutes. Of course I get tired. But I know I don't want to become the average guy. I have never seen or thought of myself as average in anything I do. And because of that I never will. I will always push myself no matter what."

Darrin knows what works for him, but the things that fuel him may not fuel your drive. Here's what he suggests for others:

"Take the time out to find out what you're passionate about and use that as your fuel. Whatever it may be it will be unique to you, even though you may have it in common with someone else. It is what will keep you going."

Your fuel can come in many forms, but whatever it is just remember, *"No one, no situation, nothing can hold you down but yourself."*

"Once you have begun to trickle into the realm of being comfortable you have given up and settled for your present state."

9
I'M COMFY SO I WILL DO IT TOMORROW

Is there ever really any benefit in waiting until tomorrow? The only thing that's really holding you back is your sheer laziness. You have the physical ability to get the job done, but you choose not to because deep down you've already given up on yourself. You feel like you can't get to the place you want to be; so, what's the point in getting up off the couch or the bed and doing something different that will only lead to no results. Well, that's not true. You can always get results. What produces "no results" is doing nothing at all. You may not see it right away, but it will come. The only thing that will prove opposite is your inability to move.

One thing that we all need to do, is a better job of realizing that tomorrow is not promised. Why would you want to put something off until tomorrow when you could easily accomplish it today? Unless you just worked out yesterday and today is your day off; there is no reason to wait. What is to stop you from doing it today? What if tomorrow never comes for you? Each day you say, *"I'll do it tomorrow"*, then you wake up and then its ten years later. You'll wonder where the time has gone and be placed in a position where it's harder to get started. By dismissing the importance of exercise through your mental state of "comfort"; you allow the result of becoming unhealthy to be an inevitable outcome when it's completely avoidable, all you have to do is start today.

Finding that inner strength can be challenging but you don't have to achieve or accomplish it alone. The power of a support system is paramount. Get a workout buddy. Those days you're feeling lazy, your workout buddy can help get you going. If not a workout buddy, then your friends and family can be your support. Let them know what you are trying to accomplish and have them hold you accountable for the goals that you set out to achieve. Keep them abreast of each step of your process, until you've reach your ultimate goal. When they see you and find you're just lying around, they can push you to get up by reminding you of your goals. Positive reinforcement can go a long way. Knowing that you have people in your corner to back you up, and pick you up when you fall can be that determining factor that keeps you going.

Just take the time out to weigh your options. Write down your goals. Right underneath that make a chart with two columns. One column should represent the positives of getting started today. The other column would represent the negatives of waiting till tomorrow. A third column is not necessary because there are no benefits of waiting until tomorrow. Once done, this will be your beginning point. This will help you see the things you want in life, along with the benefits of getting started in making that happen; including working out. Place it somewhere visible, as it will be a reminder of what you're doing and why. Use it as your motivational tool to rid yourself of the "excuse" of being comfy.

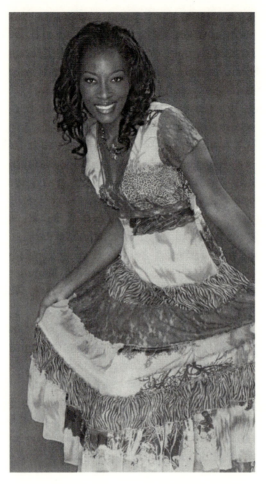

There are many ways that you can overcome staying in your comfort zone but you have to find what works for you. Once you have found that one thing that will keep you going then you will be on your way to achieve your inner greatness. You are not alone. Janice Roberson-Johnson is a Business Consultant specializing in Creative Marketing. She knows how it can be to get to comfy and not want to do things, but this proud wife and mother of two has come up with a plan to keep herself from getting to the point where she would even think this thought.

Janice chooses to work out because she knows the benefits it has.

"Working out makes me feel good. It gives me more energy and builds myself confidence. When I am consistent with my workout I feel as if I look good. I walk with a sense of self-assurance because I know that have committed myself to bettering myself."

With that in mind, she uses it to push forward to always have those feelings.

"I work out because it relieves tension and allows me to focus better."

With her being able to focus better and have less tension in her life, she is able to be better and more creative as a marketing consultant, As well as being able to focus on her family.

"The only way that I ensure this excuse doesn't prevent me from working out, is to establish a routine."

In the past when she didn't have a routine she would find herself coming up with all sorts of excuses to not get things done, and it wasn't just working out. She found that creating a routine and sticking to it worked best for her.

"I tend to work out in the mornings just before my day starts. For me, I have found this to work best; allowing me to be more consistent. Also, I think of my results, because I have experienced great results from a consistent workout schedule, I find it a bit easier to eliminate the effect of this excuse."

There have been times where a gap might occur in her schedule due to finishing a task earlier than she expected. What Janice does to compensate for the time is to begin her next task earlier, preventing herself from getting comfy.

She knows this excuse can be challenging to overcome. To help others she says,

"I would recommend that others develop a routine that works for them and stick to it. If there is a routine or workout schedule, then there will be no room for "a quick nap" or "some down-time" because this time will be scheduled and planned for working out."

This is a method that works for her. It took some time to get her routine down to where it was easy to adapt and follow but she made it happen. The key is for you to have the plan of action that best fits your lifestyle. Once you've developed your routine, you'll be on your way to achieving anything. This includes not just becoming a healthier individual, but also a more productive person.

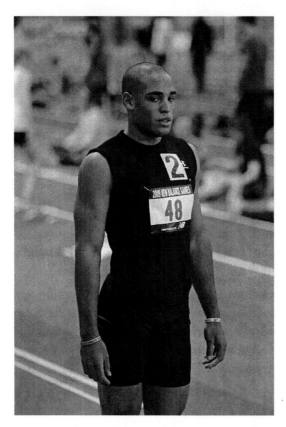

Clayton Parros, a student athlete at the University of North Carolina-Chapel Hill and also the New Jersey state record holder in the 400 meters with a time of 45.71. He knows that there is always a struggle, but finds the power and drive to succeed and get it done. His quest for achieving greatness outweighs being comfortable for a day.

We all have our own reasons and desires as to why we work out. Clayton works out because it something that has been a part of his life due to being active for the majority of his life.

"If I did not work out my life would be weird. I would feel out of place and lazy."

His desire to not feel lazy is what fuels him to continue pushing. He chose to be an athlete knowing that it would be hard work. Knowing there would be days where he would get comfortable and not feel like working out, but knew he if he wanted to be the best that it was necessary.

"Many times I will have a workout and be miserable during it;

however, afterwards I know that I have just moved one step closer to accomplishing my goal of being the best."

This focus, passion and commitment, has written his name in history. Although he recognizes that he's deserving of all the accolades, he knows it's due to all the hard work he put in on the track and weight room. I asked if he wasn't running now, or at the point when he retires, would he still exercise, here's his answer…

"…yes I would still workout and I can definitely see myself working out long after I retire. I love running so much I am going to do it as long as possible. I have been blessed with a love for running."

Hard work is something that we all know we need to do in order to achieve our goals, but for some of us we seem to let things get in the way of those goals. Clayton knows what hard work can accomplish. He is still human like the rest of us, so thoughts cross his mind often of putting off a workout till the next day but he pushes through.

"The main reasons I am able to overcome this excuse are my faith and competition."

He uses his faith and his drive for competition to keep him grounded and focused on what needs to be done. If he feels like the excuse will take over his will and drive, he'll talk to his mentors to get some extra guidance and stay focused. He understands the importance of hard work in life and competition and if he puts it off, he'll fall behind. Slacking in what he does becomes a deciding factor between a win and a loss.

"When I think about what it takes to be the best in my event and sport I know it takes constant work. I feel that I have been blessed with a gift that I need to use. I have been blessed with great successes and opportunities and I need to take advantage of them."

It's all about choices. His choice is to do what it takes regardless of what others may think or say; or if the "comfort" of laziness begins to take over, he'll fight the urge and strive to always be the best. Only you can make the choice to push through and reach your goals. No one can force you to do anything. It's important to find something that will motivate you to get up and stay up. Clayton offers this advice,

"If you have a goal work, towards it NOW! Don't put it off until later because later may never come. You never want to look back and say should have, would have or could have. DO IT!"

Don't waste time thinking about it. If you do it now you will be happier in the end.

"Creating your own excitement will lead to powerful results."

8

WORKING OUT IS TOO BORING

What makes your workout or exercising boring? Do you realize that you are in control of what you chose to do for your workouts? Since this is the case, you're the one to blame for it being boring; therefore, YOU need to make the change. Once you make the change then you won't see it as boring. Creativity is essential; you have to learn to create your own excitement in what you do. This excitement will generate the motivation to do more and produce the results you want and need.

Your workout may be boring to you because it's one dimensional and not mentally engaging or challenge to you; so you find it boring. There are ways to avoid this problem and gain some excitement to your workout. You could join a class that has student-instructor interaction such as a step aerobics class, yoga or dance class. Workouts like these require you to pay attention to the instructor and execute the movements and exercises they're asking you to perform. There are so many classes out there for you to join to gain mental stimulation as well as getting a great workout. If you can't afford to join a gym or to join group exercise classes, you can get group exercise DVDs do it on your own, with friends or even family. Schedule a time and day where everyone meets and do it together. This way you are all accountable and it helps to keep everyone involved and motivated; best of all its fun.

Another way that you could add some flair to your workouts is to create a playlist of music that incorporates different tempos. This way you can have a workout program which is tailored to the tempo of the music and base it on whatever muscles you have chosen to work out that day. This will give you variation within your workout, since you never know at what point the tempo is going to change. It'll keep you on your toes at all times because you have to be mentally prepared for the change and ready to switch gears at any point. This creative method incorporates muscle confusion which is great for achieving results. It also steers away from a monotonous routine. Keeping you more focused, motivated and excited for the next workout. Also, the music can amp you up on those moments when you want to quit, are tired or even getting a little bored. A good song can come on and you might end up telling yourself "I'll go till the end of this song", and that one song could turn into two songs and so on. Before you know it you have worked out the designated time you set out to achieve or even longer.

The best way to incorporate some cardio into your workouts is to generally find something aerobic that you enjoy. Just using stationary machinery can get boring very easily. A way to shake that up could be to take up a sport that you've always enjoyed. No matter your age there are recreation leagues for just about any type of sport for all age groups. Another option would be to just get together with friends and family and do it that way. You could take up a martial art. All martial art forms have an aerobic quality to its training program. Some are more intense than others, but they all make sure that you start off gradually. This way you won't get discouraged quickly and you will remain safe.

The key with all these suggestions is to keeping you stimulated and prevent boredom from creeping in by keeping it interesting and different. Don't knock something before you've tried it. You never know what might happen. In your skepticism, you may try a new workout regimen, group exercise program or video and fall in love with it. Get other people to do it with you. Friends and family are a good place to start, but even finding someone you don't know who shares similar issues could be beneficial. The two of you can find a way to make it more creative and fun, as well push each other. Sometimes two heads are better than one.

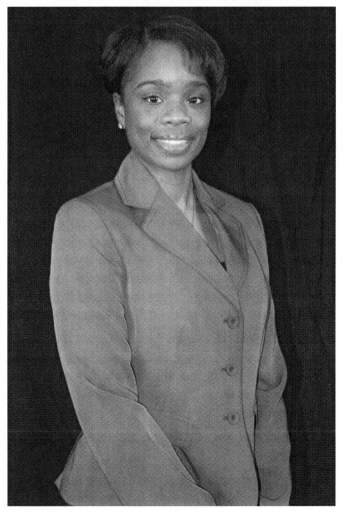

Here's a woman who finds different ways to keep herself engaged while working out. She finds different ways to keep it interesting and fun at the same time.

Anna Johnson, licensed real estate consultant and Investor, and mother. Even though she has a demanding schedule she always makes time to exercise.

When asked why she works out she replied by saying,

"I workout because I know how important it is to my health. High blood pressure and high cholesterol run in the family. I am also the

smallest person in my immediate and extended family. Everyone is BIG!!! So there is a high probability to be big, have high blood pressure and high cholesterol. I don't want that for myself. I want to live a long time. That motivates me to keep it together and focus on my workout. I also love the way I feel afterwards. I have lots of energy. If I had a bad day, working out always makes me feel much better. It relieves the stress of the day. I also workout for vanity reasons, I like to look good in my clothes and naked and working out makes my body look great."

She finds different things in her life to fuel her drive to exercise. Realizing that there are different things that she could fall victim to pushes her that much harder.

The excuse of being bored is easy to use for most people but Anna finds ways to keep it from holding her back.

"I do not allow boredom to hold me back from exercising because I am constantly thinking of different ways of challenging myself and keeping it interesting. If I get bored, I won't do it. For instance, I find the treadmill very boring so I don't do it at all. Instead I take spin class. It burns tons of calories; we listen to great music and its fun. Last year I took tennis lessons, after three lessons I quit because I was bored."

Anna engages in the activities she loves to remove the boredom out of her workout. She has taken different dance classes from Caribbean to Hip Hop. She found herself having lots of fun while doing the classes, and it was keeping her in great shape. She's also trained for and finished a half marathon for a charity.

"I was very motivated because I thought of the sickly individuals that I was running for."

Her methods of preventing to success is finding things she enjoys and sticking with those. Here's what she suggests to people who find themselves saying that working out is boring.

"What I would suggest to people would be first, tell people about your workout goals. When you know that people are watching you, it keeps you accountable and you will work harder to meet those goals. I would also suggest that you get a workout partner or a group. Workout with friends because it's fun and it really motivates you to keep going and they push you to work harder even if you want to give up. You also don't want to let them down if you don't show up. You rely on each other."

If this doesn't work, she suggests,

"...[do] an activity that you love. People tend to stick with something if they like what they're doing. Join a class that you will enjoy such as dancing, biking, boxing, yoga, pole dancing, and step aerobics, anything that interest you. This will make it more fun and take the boredom out. You will actually look forward to working out."

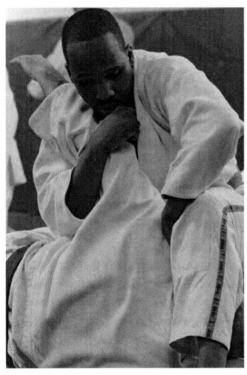

Tairie Sanders, a banker at Bank of America; used to find working out to be very boring. Now it has become part of his lifestyle. He describes how he prevented this excuse from holding him back.

Growing up Tairie was always into athletics and martial arts. A former high school and collegiate track runner, prior to him ending his athletic career he had *already achieved a 1st degree black belt in Tai Kwon Do and a purple belt in Ninjutsu. Once his athletic career was over he didn't workout because he felt it was boring and anytime he would begin, he'd stop shortly after. He finally realized that there was more to working out besides just looking good.* When asked what's different now he gave this answer.

"I workout for many reason but the most important I would say is physical fitness, just overall to stay healthy. I can't lie there is also the incentive to be a little bit more attractive to the opposite sex, I mean come on if I take of my shirt and have six pack abs like Usher I really don't think any woman would tell me to put my shirt back on, lol"

He also said,

"Just wanting to stay healthy keeps me working hard. Martial arts was always very fun for me, so to avoid being bored I started back with

martial arts again. I began with Brazilian Jiu-Jitsu. It helped me excel a lot faster and kept me interested. The desire to excel at something I love is what keeps me going to stay working out; I also worked out with a personal trainer for some time to help to increase my strength. He made it fun and showed me that it's not always a boring chore."

Although Tairie had begun to find working out boring, he found ways to make it fun and exciting and used something he loved to his advantage. Since he was able to overcome this excuse, he provided the following advice.

"I used to find it boring, so to avoid beginning and failing again I went back to doing something I loved. With that initial start it allowed me to be more inviting to other forms of exercise. With that I hired a trainer to show me how to train properly and keep it fun for me so that I can continue to do it. Not to mention it helped me out a lot when it came to my Brazilian Jiu-Jitsu."

He's gotten himself so focused that boredom isn't an option for him any longer. Health has become a priority in his life because of this; it keeps him pressing forward to be better at everything he does.

"I usually don't find excuses to miss a workout. Although life sometimes gets in the way, I get out of work late and I really don't want to go to the gym this late. I would say 90% of the time I still go and work out but the other 10% of the time if I don't go I feel guilty, which is a good sign that I know that working out means a lot to me."

Tairie believes if you find a reason to make your exercise regimen mean more than just working out, you won't create excuses to avoid it.

"I would suggest to people to be like Nike 'just do it', just do something in your life. We only get one shot; there is no pause rewind or fast forward. So the healthier you are usually means the longer you will have to enjoy life. I would say just get started and slowly work into it. Don't just go to the gym workout like a mad man or mad women for a month and then quit because you don't see results."

It is important to set deliverables to achieve your ultimate health and fitness goals. This will serve as a positive reinforcement to keep yourself going. The more positive reinforcement you have the more likely you are to stick with it. Finding something you enjoy doing and giving yourself deliverables will go a long way.

Here are some of Tairie's final thoughts.

"Look at working out like an ice sculpting an artist would a big block of ice. In the beginning it doesn't look like anything, then he slowly methodically starts chipping away patiently and with care and before you know it there is a beautiful work of art. I say the body is just like that, you may not see your flat stomach or six pack abs but it is there under all that fat. You just have to be patient and methodical about chipping it away. Then just like the block of ice you will be a beautiful work of art inside and out"

"Going the extra mile and doing some extra can go a long way to endless possibilities. Anything less would limit your true potential."

7

I ALREADY GET ENOUGH EXERCISE

D o you think that what you already do in your life is enough? Well you're wrong! There is a rapidly growing misconception that your regular daily activity is enough and you don't have to do more than that. Why the misconception? Simply because there is still a need to maintain the level of activity that you currently have in your life. Much like a student who has to continuously study to maintain the good grades that they are getting; the studying is their "exercise" of the mind. In order to stay functional, you have to do something extra in order to maintain and that extra comes in the form of exercise.

Have you ever wondered why, even with all your activity, you still find yourself getting tired or out of breath just walking up stairs. Well, it's because the body adapts quickly. Just because you are doing things which keep you active doesn't mean you're getting enough exercise. That may sound strange to some people, but if you continue any activity with consistency your body will begin to plateau. The exercise you do may cause you to work up a sweat or elevate your heart rate, but because you're doing constant similar repetition you will see no physical change. This is why, lately, there has been an increased emphasis on what's called muscle confusion. Your workout should do just what the name implies - *confuse* your muscles! Why would you want to confuse your muscles, you may ask? The answer is; to keep them in a constant state of development. Think of it like being in a classroom. In order to stay engaged in something you're learning, you have to constantly be challenged otherwise you lose concentration. The same happens in your body. By using muscle confusion techniques you can continuously keep your body engaged, "learn something new" and prevent it from reaching a plateau. The easiest and simplest way to achieve this is to vary your workout. Something that simple can help you to start seeing changes. Whether it's exercising to workout your body or your mind; you need to be willing to push further in order to maintain and increase productivity. No matter who you are, you can benefit from this idea in some way. So when thinking that what you are doing is enough, remember just a little extra effort can create so much more in your life.

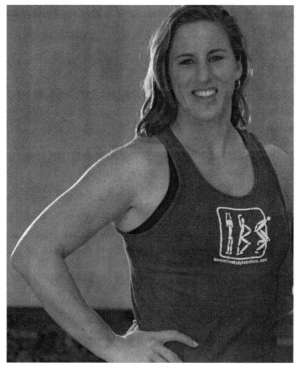

This woman has no choice to be active because what she does for a living involves her using her body to accomplish the work. It's physically demanding, but she still makes time to get in the extra exercise. Find out why.

Anne Tierney, co-creator of Ki-Hara Resistance Stretching. She teaches her stretching techniques to personal clients, as well as other instructors who'd like to use it with their clients. There are lots of people who believe what they do during the course of the day should suffice for not working out, but they're wrong. The body adapts to repetitive actions, or closely related actions. What you assume is working your body out, might not be doing as much as you may think. In Anne's case, her line of work forces her to use a lot of her body and muscles; creating the resistance for each of the stretch used and still makes it her business to workout. Working out is a very large portion of her life. Anne was involved in sports at a young age. She went on to compete as a collegiate athlete and became an Academic All-American basketball player. Despite all her accomplishments as an athlete and her profession, she continues to workout.

"I like working out…it helps to keep me in shape, relieve my stress and keep me healthy. I would still work out if I was doing something else. I used to work in corporate America and it was even more important then."

An overall good level health and well-being is her motivation to exercise.

What keeps this excuse from not holding her back, is the fact that she knows the importance of keeping balance in the body for both strength and flexibility.

"I have to exercise to keep my strength up and keep me healthy because my line of work is so demanding on my body."

She doesn't workout for anyone else but for herself. This makes it easier for her to avoid distractions which would keep her from working out and or making excuses. Although she puts demands on her body all day to train others, she doesn't allow that to stop her.

"There is no greater stress relief than working out on my own."

Exercise can definitely aid in the reduction of stress relief. It's just an added bonus for her since it's something she already loves. Of course, there have been times where it has crossed her mind – after a long exhausting day – to reconsider her daily workout; however, she maintains her personal goals and benefits, sucks it up, and pushes through a workout.

Helping others is a part of Anne's nature. She has a passion to help others which is why she does what she does. Since she likes to help people, I asked her for some tips for people who may find themselves feeling as if they've done enough; she says,

"Stay determined and have fun."

If you can stay determined and focused on your goals, you will have no problems fighting the temptation to take days off or fall victim to this or any other excuse. Anne also says,

"In order to maintain what you have at minimum, you always have to do a little something extra to keep you leveled."

Variety is important, try not to get caught up in doing the same thing all the time.

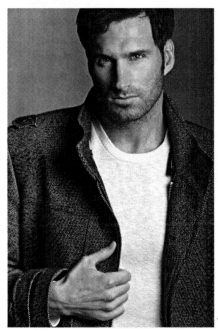

Here's another person who gets a lot of exercise from their profession and still makes time to get in some extra exercise in order to maintain a healthy lifestyle, and strong body. Neil Andrews, personal trainer for 14 years and model for 9 years.

Despite having ties to the health and wellness field, he still works out on his own. Regardless of his ties to this profession, he would still workout.

"Exercise has been such a big part of my life long before I started to do any of these things. I realized the great benefits I feel and receive from a healthy lifestyle and way of living and how strong and vibrant I feel every day. Exercise is just a very important part of life, no matter who you are. It is like owning a car. You need to service the engine to keep it running properly. Exercise is the same in that it helps your body to run at its best. Without it your body is not performing to its highest level regardless of your age or gender."

Neil's reasons for working out go even deeper than that.

"I exercise because it is good for my mind and body. By strengthening

my body I know that my body will continue to serve as a strong tool for my day to day life as I continue to get older. Mentally it helps me to feel great and alert. I also like to work out because it is fun and I enjoy doing it. I also want to look good and I want to be able to look back upon my life and be proud of the accomplishments I have made with my body with the way it looks and feels."

Exercise can also help reduce the risk of diseases, and help individuals maintain a healthy strong posture to perform day to day activities with ease. When it comes to exercise, there is no lack of focus with Neil. He doesn't let much deter him.

"I know the important of exercise regardless of your age, race, or gender. Since lack of exercise will causes your muscles to atrophy or shrink and weaken I can't take that chance, I on the other hand like to be challenged and from experience know when I need more or less exercise. Without my body being healthy I have nothing and cannot go about my life with confidence and ease because I would feel weak. So that is a factor into realizing I need to continue to always exercise and sweat."

This is how he keeps himself from falling victim to this excuse.

If someone feels they've gotten enough exercise and are healthy and strong then good for them that may not always be true.

"Everyone has the same 24 hours in the day. I understand that people have different factors of time constraints such as work, family, kids, etc. but everyone has the same 24 hours and the right to choose how to live their lives."

Being aware of your time and learning how to manage it can help you make things happen. You just need to truly want it before so that it can come. Neil also says,

"So many people need reality checks and [should] honestly ask the question, am I happy with myself, health and body? I guarantee most people can find at least 15-30 minutes in their day to do some kind of acrobic or strength activity such as body weights, squats, walking, crunches or pushups from their own home. You don't need a lot of equipment or know how. You just got to start moving and keep moving. At least you are doing something and not sitting around."

Neil says it best, if you want it, it will come!

"The ability to find happiness and greatness within you can avoid the demise of compliments in the form of distractions."

6 MY SIGNIFICANT OTHER/ LOVED ONES LIKE ME THE WAY THAT I AM

I guess I could see how this could be an excuse, but at the same time another's thoughts shouldn't change the fact that you need to be happy with yourself, as well as healthy. We all strive to make those closest to us as happy and proud of us. When those who we care about give us these "compliments", it can be a great distraction from really paying attention to the greater need to remain healthy. There is such a thing as physically appearing to be healthy on the outside, and being the exact opposite on the inside. How many times have we heard of someone who became ill, terminally ill or died; and we thought to ourselves "Wow I didn't even know they were sick, they looked fine to me." This happens because your body is a whole and you have to take care of it as such. Yes, we all want to look good for our significant other or when attending family functions, but the true "compliment" would be to remain healthy and gain total wellness.

When you receive these compliments, you can use them as motivational tools to help you remain that way and keep the compliments coming. Instead of one day being in a position where the compliments stop and turn to questions of, "what happened to you", among those same family and friends. To prevent this from happening, focus yourself on continuing to look good so that the "compliments" or comments don't change. Your true friends and family will always love you no matter what, but that doesn't mean they don't love the way you look and want you to continue to look that way. Even if you get the infamous question from them "why are you going to workout you don't need to?" Just smile and reply, "I am going because I want to continue to look this good as well as continue to have good health so I can be around a long time for you to enjoy me". You can remind them that they don't want to wake up one day and you're not there anymore. This can become a harsh but true reality based on how rapidly a person's health can decline without the proper precautions being taken.

Many people fall victim to trying to please people in their life, such as their significant other, but don't think about what they need to do for themselves in order to remain happy. People need to realize that you have to be happy with yourself before you can truly be happy with someone else. This lack of "self-happiness" can create other complications within your relationships, work ethic and just the ability to do everyday things. The benefits from exercise vary, but that of looking good and feeling good is probably at the top of the list. So why would you want to avoid being able to look good and feel good? Where is the benefit in that? If you can't find a benefit in it then it shouldn't be your starting point

A tip to help you to stay motivated when getting positive compliments is to have your significant other to join you for a workout. This way the two of you are doing it together, keeping each other motivated and focused; no one is holding the other back from getting it done. If they do not have the desire to work out like you do, then you can just let them know that this is something that you want and need their support; and with their support you can achieve your goals, and by achieving your goals you both can be happy together, ultimately reducing the conflict in your relationship. Besides, who doesn't want less conflict in their lives? Less conflict means less stress, and stress can lead to weight gain. The lower your stress levels, the better you would be mentally and physically.

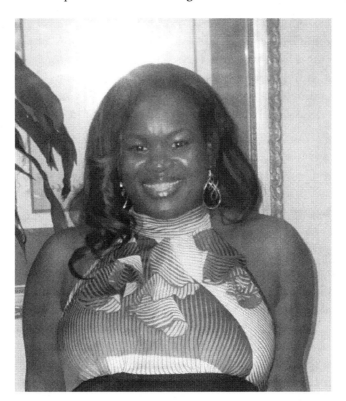

Here's the story of a woman who finds it within herself to workout, despite the positive compliments she receives from her husband and loved ones. This is an account of her focus and determination.

Tali' Morgan-Hughes, Information Technology Change Manager, mother of two, wife, daughter, best friend and mentor. She is also in school working on her degree and despite all of this; she still has the desire to exercise. When asked why she exercises even though she doesn't have to, she responded by saying,

"I choose to exercise to clear my mind and keep my spirit vibrant. Everyday life can bring situations in which you can't control. Exercising grants me the ability to take control and push myself for an hour or more by doing some form of physical activity. Exercising provides me the ability to reflect on me. Maintaining a healthy lifestyle is critical for me to continue to be a factor in my family and friends lives. I exercise since improving the shape of my body is a goal I set for myself. Once the goal is obtained I will continue to exercise and maintain the body investment I have worked towards. Exercising is an investment for my body."

She also feels that if she doesn't workout it would jeopardize her overall health and put herself in a predicament where she can become ill over the bad foods she chose to eat, in addition to the lack of exercise. It doesn't just stop there. Tali' receives the compliments from her husband and family, and still continues to workout despite consistently told she looks great and there's no need. I asked her why she continues to do so, her response,

> *"I don't exercise to please family or friends. I exercise because it is a lifestyle choice I have decided to incorporate into the healthy life I want to live. The positive feedback I receive only motivates me to continue on working towards sculpting my body into what I want it to be and maintaining the figure I want. Exercising shouldn't be about pleasing anyone but you. You are the most important motivator to continue on taking charge of your body."*

Although she accepts the positive feedback she receives from her family and friends, she simply uses it to increase the motivation she already has to workout and maintain a healthy lifestyle. It is who she chose to be. This is powerful because there are many who will get comfortable with their situation and fall short of striving to be better than the day they were before and maintain.

When asked what suggestions she would have for someone reading this book and leaning the excuses listed here as well as others, Tali' said,

> *"Take ownership of wanting to exercise for YOU. Make and take time out of your day to incorporate sometime of physical activity into your daily routine. It's a responsibility everyone should own. Don't let compliments or excuses dictate that exercising should halt once a goal is obtained. Exercising is not only about reaching a goal but maintaining the results. Think of exercising as a building that should never collapse. This means maintaining and reconstruction where need can never cease. Exercising will stabilize and keep the body strong no matter the age. "*

Tali' has found what works for her but you have to find out what works best for you. These are just suggestions to help prevent this from holding you back. You have the power to make the change. Just find out what is important to you and use that as a focus. If you want to be able to continue to be there for your significant other and loved ones, it will start by you taking care of yourself first.

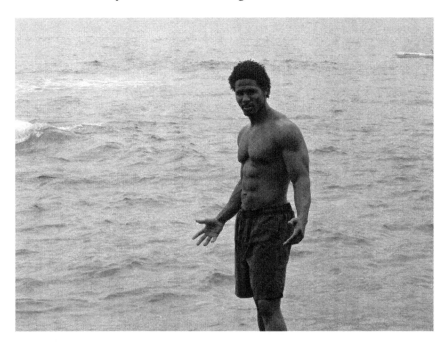

This next gentleman has been there and done that when it comes to this excuse. He was in a relationship where his significant other would get upset because he would choose to go workout instead of spend time with her. At times he would fall victim, but he had to find the strength and the focus to make sure that he stuck to his goals and dreams.

Luther Bowen, High School football coach. Coach Bowen – as the kids call him – is a wide receiver coach and also one of the offensive coordinators. Luther had many different reasons for exercising throughout his life. Depending on when you talked to him would depend on his purpose of why he worked out. However, one thing that never changed was his desire to always be healthy. That was his foundation. After that, the rest was just extra motivation and drive to prepare him for what he wanted. He says,

"I work out because it has become a part of my life. If I don't work out one day I feel weak, tired, and sluggish and basically like a bum."

He worked out because he was a collegiate and professional football player in the Arena Football League. However, his profession didn't stop him from also wanting to be in shape for aesthetic reasons.

"I'm always trying to better myself and stay physically fit. I like how I feel when I'm in shape and I like to have a sexy body for the ladies."

Luther believes at the age of 60, it will time to stop working out so hard.

> *"I always tell people when I'm 60 I'm going to let it go. There is no reason why I'm going to be in the weight room at 60 trying to kill myself, but I always think that I'm going to do some sort of cardio. Maybe a light jog because that's how you keep your body healthy."*

Even he knows at the age of 60 that he will still do some sort of exercise and activity even if it's not lifting heavy weights.

People often set fitness and exercise goals for the wrong reasons. This tends to be the reason or "cause" as to why people fall short or let a particular excuse hold them back from what they may truly want. When it comes to priorities he feels,

> *"It's not about what my partner feels. It's about what I feel and if I feel I don't look good then I'm going to work out."*

Luther's self-esteem is what prevents him from being hindered by excuses and stopping from him getting where he wants to be. Of course every once in a while he will skip a workout to make sure that his partner is happy, but he also works out to help his partner understand how important it is to him and how it makes him happy. For him to be happy with her he first needs to be happy with himself. Luther also tells his partner,

> *"If you are happy with the way that I look now then I have to continue to work hard to make sure that I stay looking good the way you like you right now."*

By reinforcing the reasons why he works out in the first place, it establishes the connection they have and helps his partner to understand that if she enjoys what she sees, he has to maintain it. He'd also bring her to workout with him.

> *"I would bring her with me to the gym as a reminder of how much she likes how I look and to see me sweat."*

When asked for tips and/or suggestions for others who may run into a similar situation with their significant other he says,

> *"I would tell someone your partner is probably lying to you because they don't want you to feel bad, or they just got comfortable with your body. But it's always good to impress them or to surprise them with a new look. You may be used to your car but if someone bought you a new Bentley you would like it and drive it."*

Including your significant other in your life and routine will go a long way in getting them to understand and be supportive of what it is that you want for you. It might even get them motivated to do the same, if they aren't already.

"Finding the connection of importance to one's self is the key to success, focus and continued motivation in life."

5 I'M NOT MOTIVATED

Out of all the excuses this is one that probably gets to me the most. The reason is because it just boggles my mind that you could really convince yourself that you have no motivation to begin an exercise program. In my opinion, it goes deeper than just beginning an exercise program. It's a lack of motivation for living a long and healthy life. What could be more important than for you to have motivation to stay alive? No matter what you want to do in life and no matter what goals and aspirations you would like to achieve, none will be able to be accomplished without having the good health to see them through.

Having knowledge of the consequences of not incorporating exercise into your life can also be a way that you could motivate yourself; on the other hand, knowing that you could increase your life expectance should also be a motivating factor. Think about it. What if you had knowledge that your quality of life could possibly suffer if you didn't begin to do something soon? The things that you enjoy doing now or things that you have plans to do in the future may not happen. If you have children, could not being able to play with them change your stance about having lack of motivation? Could you imagine not being able to complete simple things around the house due to being overweight, as well as becoming fatigued very easily? Not to mention all of the other health risks you invite into your life; all because you *believe* you can't find the motivation to get up and get started.

Motivation comes from within you. No one can force you to do anything you truly don't want to do, and because of this factor; no matter how much someone tries to get you to do something it has to be up to you to make the choice to do it. The help of others can get you motivated and help you stay focused; in addition to moving in the right direction with anything in life. The power of having an "exercise buddy" or friends to help you with any goals you have in life is great. This increases the accountability factor because now you have someone or a group of people that will keep you on your toes and vice versa. When there are times where you don't feel motivated to work out, you have someone who can say come on "let's do it". In the end, it will help you get and stay motivated.

A way of getting yourself motivated is by setting goals, but you have to set *S.M.A.R.T.* goals. S.M.A.R.T. stands for *S*pecific, *M*easurable, *A*ttainable, *R*ealistic and *T*imely. Setting these types of goals leaves less room for discouragement. If you have a large goal to achieve but don't set a specific plan to get there, you will quit due to lack of planning. It's not that the goal was unattainable, but because you didn't yourself a *specific, measurable, attainable* and *realistic* way to there, within a *timely* fashion. Goal setting and planning is the key to success. Knowing where you want to be is just the beginning; but creating the plan to get there is the way to keep you motivated.

A self assessment is a great way to get you going in conjunction with your S.M.A.R.T. goals. Here is a simple yet effective self assessment form which can help guide you to achieve your goals.

Self Assessment

The following questions will help determine your level of readiness to make lifestyle changes, your motivation towards reaching your goals, and identifying obstacles to your success. There is no right or wrong answers to these questions. The information you write down will be used to help you in your development to get started into the right direction.

- Are you placing your health at risk because of your current behaviors or lifestyle? If so, please describe. (ex. smoking, drug use, sedentary, overweight, etc)

- Are you seeking to make lifetime changes or reach a short-term, temporary goal?

- Are you open to trying different approaches or do you have preferred methods, areas to avoid, etc?

- Are you willing to set realistic goals and prepared to deal with possible setbacks?

- Are you willing to make lifestyle changes or would you rather maintain your current lifestyle with slight modifications?

- Have you made previous attempts at lifestyle changes? If so, what were the results?

- Compared to previous attempts, how motivated are you at this time to try to change your lifestyle? (1-5 scale; 1=not at all motivated, 5= extremely motivated)

- Are there outside factors (work, family, travel, etc) that could impact your ability to make lifestyle changes? If so, list:

- How confident are you that you can work regular exercise into your daily schedule starting tomorrow? (use a 1-5 scale; 1=not at all confident, 5=extremely confident)

- Indicate your busiest day of the week and your easiest day of the week.
- Busiest: _____
- Easiest: _____

- List any challenges that are a result of your present situation (e.g., "none of my clothes fit"; "I have no energy"; "My blood pressure is too high").

- Are you looking for improvements in:
- weight _____
- appearance _____
- health _____
- energy _____
- injury recovery _____
- other _____

A few tips that may help you get going when losing motivation are:
1. *Doing something fun*
2. *Doing something that isn't so complicated*
3. *Doing something that is relaxing to your body.*

Doing something fun can consist of anything. It doesn't have to be lifting weights or running on a treadmill to be considered exercise. If you like to dance you can go out dancing. It can be just that simple as long as your active it's actually exercise. Doing something less complicated helps because it makes it seem as if it's not hard to do. When something is a little easier, you find yourself wanting to do more of it and frequently. Lastly, you can choose to do something that is relaxing to your body. Just because its exercise doesn't mean it can't make you feel good. Doing something like yoga is a form of exercise that is designed to give your body a soothing and relaxing sensation, while working it at the same time. Finding balance and creating variety can help you get and stay motivated.

Discovering your relevance…your purpose in this life and that key aspect to focus on is what will get you to begin thinking about the future, as opposed to only thinking about the here and now. There is more to life than just what is in front of you. Thinking about and only acting for the present is great, but don't you want to be able to enjoy it for years to come?

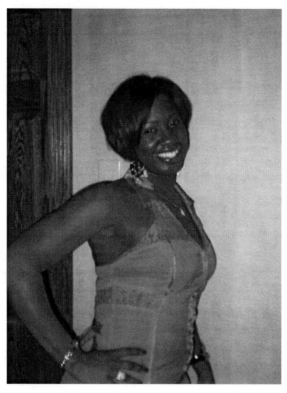

This next woman does not have to work out and could easily find reasons to not be motivated, but doesn't. She draws her motivation from things deep within her and the desire to always be better is what moves her.

Natasha Quarles, Ultrasound Technician. Motivation is defined as the state or condition of being motivated. What motivates Natasha is the desire to excel. Her motivation for working out is to excel at keeping herself healthy. She says,

"I enjoy working out because it gives me a lot of energy and I love the way my body looks after a good work out."

Who doesn't want to look great all the time and have a mental state that's always positive, free and clear?

"I work out because I love the way my clothes look on me. I love the wardrobe I have now. I like to shop, but I'd rather save money by

keeping my body tight the way it is now and not have to go out and continuously buy new clothing due to weight gain. "

Ultimately she enjoys the fact that it makes her feel good overall.

"I always try to make it enjoyable that helps to keep me motivated so I stick with it. If that doesn't work I get a personal trainer to help keep me focused and on task to stick with my plan."

Since she has the desire to achieve, she doesn't let this excuse hold her back. Nothing could be worse than not achieving the goals which she has set for herself physically and mentally, but also in life overall.

"Since I keep my work outs enjoyable and with the help of a trainer I can have a variation which helps to keep me motivated. As well as enjoying the results that working out brings and the overall feel good experience is enough to not let myself fall victim to this excuse."

Too many of us don't even realize how many motivating things that we have in our lives that we overlook. In reality it could be something very small that you could focus on and have it be a major driving force, enabling you to do anything you want in life. Natasha has her own set of motivating factors that prevent her from falling victim to this excuse.

"Being able to wake up in the morning and look in the mirror and like the way I feel and look is enough to keep me from using this excuse. I weigh my options and the benefits are just greater than the excuse itself, therefore it's not an excuse for me."

Anything is attainable as long as you try. So what can you do to keep yourself motivated? First, you need to figure out what you would like to do and then make a plan to do so. Being aware of what you can handle can help you to stay motivated and get to where you want to be. Natasha adds,

"A healthy heart is something that will last you a lifetime, only if you keep it health. Think about that when you come up with an excuse to not get your work out in."

There are so many things you can do. Just believe in yourself and have fun.

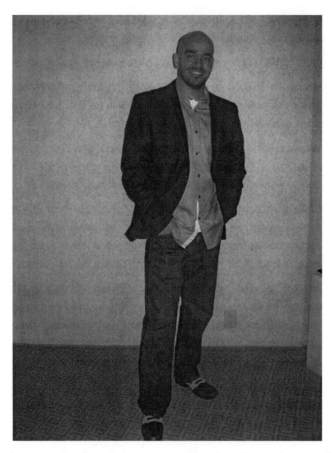

Here's a guy who doesn't have to workout but does it because he wants to and finds reasons to motivate him. Motivation has to be found from within and he sure has found it for himself.

Russell Battle, Information Technology Network Specialist for IBM. Everyone has their own reasons for working out. Russell had many reasons for why he works out. When asked to narrow it down to his top three he said,

> *"I work out because I want to stay health first and foremost, I want to gain more muscle and I want to make sure that I look great naked."*

He wants to make sure that he stays healthy because he would like to live long and be able to enjoy his family when he has one. He doesn't want to get older and have his body age more rapidly than his years on this Earth, so in the future when he decides to have kids he'll be able to run around, jump and play with them.

"I like to work out and I enjoy the results that I see after I am finished. I also like the compliments I get about the way that I look. Being able to stay away from having more visits to the doctor besides an annual checkup is always a plus."

Russell is not shy; he's vocal about his wants and has no problem speaking it into existence.

"Majority of people would love to look great naked they may just phrase it differently. I know what I want so I just say it and once it's said I put in my mind a plan of action on how I am going to achieve that goal."

Russell sets the goals to be achieved and places it in his mind to accomplish them. Once his mind is made up there is no stopping him. This is how he keeps his motivation, making his goals visible also helps sustain his drive.

"If I can see them and I know that I haven't hit them, then it only gives me more fuel to add to my fire to make sure it gets accomplished."

Staying motivated isn't always an easy task but you have to find it deep within your mind and body to want it bad enough. Once you find it no one can take it away from you.

"…if you keep in mind why you're working out and make sure the work outs are effective, you will see results which will keep you motivated. Also, make sure you stay consistent."

Consistency is the key to reaching new heights. Whatever level you want, it can be attained. Create and post on a goal board. Check off each goal when you achieve them. Maybe even create a competition with friends or family, have a prize for the winner. These are just examples of ways you can prevent lack of motivation. Ultimately you have to find what works for you.

4 I DON'T WANT TO GET MY HAIR MESSED UP

ontrary to popular belief, this excuse isn't just used by women. There are men who fear working out will ruin their hair, too. Oddly enough you chose the hairstyle; no one else. It can also be your choice to pick a hairstyle more conducive to exercising. Another option is learning more about at-home hair care and researching waterless (spray) shampoos, which conveniently cleanse the hair between shampoos or after any activity that dirties your strands.

Even more rewarding is engaging in a physical activity you love despite its effect on your hair. However, many people have a convoluted way of prioritizing what's important in their lives and will avoid their favorite activities because of a high-maintenance hairstyle. For example, if someone offered you a monetary reward or a something valuable in exchange for participating in a physical activity that would wreak havoc on your hair, you'd probably do it anyway. Why? Many people desire material things and direct their focus toward another's perception of themselves; however, being healthier and fit can increase your self-esteem and improve the way you're viewed.

For some of you, an attractive hairstyle is an essential part of self-esteem and pride, but how good would it feel to have a great body and improved health to match your coif? Most people don't realize that neglecting your body can actually cause hair damage. Now, the perfect hairstyle you've strived to achieve lays lifeless and limp because your body lacks nutrients and is in overall poor health. This can happen because you chose to avoid exercise, a simple task with so many benefits. Take the time to think about what's important to you and see how not taking care of your body can impact your hair's appearance. Maybe you'll figure out a way to make it work for you.

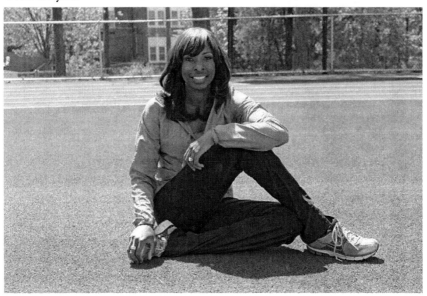

Don't just take my words. Listen to this three-time Olympian, who doesn't hair hold her back from doing what she does best.

Hazel Clark, Nike Professional Runner, six-time national champ, three-time Olympian and an Olympic finalist. Hazel works hard to be the best athlete in her event which is the 800-meter race. She says,

"I workout because I want to be the best and retain my endorsement deals by performing well,"

One would assume that the only reason this hardworking woman exercises is because she has to, but that's not the whole story. She says,

"If I wasn't a professional athlete I would do Pilates, yoga and strength

training. But I will not sweat out my hairstyles! Just joking, but there will be no more five- mile runs!"

She knows the importance of being in great health and shape, as well as the benefits of a fit body.

"When my career is over some say I won't work out, but I do like being healthy and the way working out makes my body feel and look. I will make sure I do some form of exercise and eat well to keep myself healthy at all times."

As a woman who runs for a living, you'd think Hazel wouldn't be concerned with her hair, but that's an assumption. She wears her own hair as much as possible, and says it makes her feel free. While she has always likes to look cute; Hazel's competitive nature makes the appearance of her hair a secondary concern.

"My hate of losing outweighs my desire to have cute hairstyles. Despite all of that I still hate leaving the beauty parlor knowing I'm only going to sweat out my hair."

Between salon visits, Hazel wears versatile; yet, protective hairstyles that don't require lots of heat.

"I use weaves and braids because they allow you to blow-dry and flat iron your hair after a workout and still look good. I also throw a wide headband on for a neat look. I tell myself I can be cute in the off season with my medal around my neck."

Like Hazel, find a goal that drives you. For some people this could be something so simple as looking great on the beach. Let goals like this motivate you to ignore a few bad hair days in the fall, winter and spring.

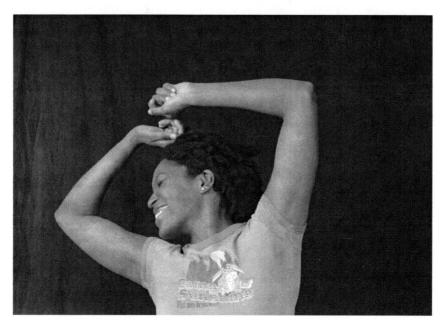

Another active woman, Veronica Davis, doesn't let her natural hair hinder her demanding workouts. Veronica is a self-employed partner and principal planner at Nspiregreen LLC, a sustainability solutions consulting company. Veronica chooses to work out because,

> *"...it is important to longevity and reduction of health risks later in life."*

While incorporating exercise into her routine makes Veronica look good on the outside, it also makes her feel good on the inside and improves her health in the long-term

> *"I am aware that I'm predisposition to some serious diseases. While I can't control my DNA, I can control my lifestyle."*

The fitness buff uses words from people she knows and quotes and anecdotes to stay focused and motivated. One of her favorite sayings is, *"Genetics loads the gun, but environment pulls the trigger."*

> *There are lots of women who may think they fall victim to the "hair excuse"; but on the contrary, maintaining a natural style can be simple. Veronica's natural hairstyle allows her to wear many different looks, she says,*

> *"Most of the styles that I wear can survive a week of sweating at the*

gym...I can say as a result of working out and eating healthy, my hair is healthy."

Veronica chose to find a hairstyle that accommodates her active lifestyle, now you have to decide what's most important to you; how good your hair looks or how good your body feels.

"Just because you don't have the answer right in front of you, doesn't mean it can't be found."

3 I DON'T KNOW WHAT TO DO

Why are you so afraid to ask for some help if you don't know what to do? There are so many resources to find different ways to work out, exercises for each muscle group, and even different ways to have healthier eating habits. Your resources include the people in your life, your doctor, a bookstore, and the easiest...the internet. There's tons of information on the internet that can help you to accomplish anything; including creating a workout regime. Most of us already spend time doing other things on the internet; so dedicating a little bit of that time and energy to search for things that can help you achieve your fitness goals, wouldn't hurt. Furthermore, most of us at least have one person in our lives who is health conscious or who works out, whether they're an exercise fanatic or even if they just do it for general health; you know them. They would be more than willing to assist you in learning what to do and finding out what will work for you. These people are always looking for friends to join them in working out and eating right so they don't have to do it alone. This way you can support each other.

All of those examples come are of no cost to you. Even if you belong to a gym, there are fitness professionals there who can assist you if you just ask. If you're unsure about something all you have to do is ask. Verbal advice from one of the fitness professionals at your gym is always free of charge. Alternatively, if you need the help of someone to keep you motivated or focused on achieving your goals, you can employ the help of a personal trainer or a nutritionist to help guide and work with your weight loss goals. The price of these services can vary based on what exactly you're looking for and how long. However, it is not something that is mandatory for you to achieve your goals; there are many free options available much like the ones listed above. There are even many health, wellness and fitness magazines out there that offer different exercise ideas, and sometimes even sample work out regimens that you can follow. Subscriptions to these magazines are available at affordable rates. There are also books and DVD's that you can purchase to help you get the information you're looking for to achieve your goals.

Most of us at minimum have heard of pushups, jumping jacks, sit-ups, crunches etc. At some point in our lives – whether it was gym class or something similar – we had to perform these exercises. So in actuality you do know some where you can start. Getting started is probably the hardest part, but once your started you will be fine. If you start with just those simple exercises and do them for 10-20 minutes a day, you will soon see changes in your body. Then at that point you will be able to graduate to more advanced exercises and regimens. The key is to just ask or search for your answers on what to do. If you never begin there, then you will always feel like you don't know what to do. You have a basic knowledge of where to start because as kids those simple exercises were instilled in us. Finding out what to do is easy. Just get it done.

To give you more of an understanding of this is a young woman who had her share of road blocks but didn't let it stop her from finding an answer. She stayed focused and wasn't about to let anything stop her.

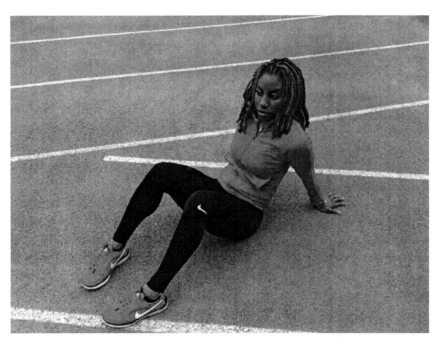

Janine Davis, graduate assistant (GA) and Assistant Coach for The State University of Rutgers -Newark Track & Field team, graduate student in their Master of Arts in Public Administration program, as well as assistant to 4-time Olympian Joetta Clark Diggs – Founder and Executive Director of the Joetta Clark Diggs Sports Foundation.

Janine had a reason to work out for a large portion of her life. So it was just a part of what she did through her daily or weekly routines. Not only was she on scholarship, she was also a division one collegiate track & field athlete. Exercise, as well as strong academics, was mandatory during her college years. She says,

> *"All of the elements that came with that package gave me no room to miss a day of training, so I had no choice."*

But eventually she had to graduate and her collegiate career was over. After her last race she took off and decided to do nothing. No running no lifting or any exercise at all.

> *"After a summer of letting myself go, I started to see my muscle tone go and my energy level drop. This inspired me to get back on some kind of workout regimen."*

Janine realizing that exercise wasn't just part of her collegiate career, it was part of her lifestyle, sparked a surge of motivation and inspiration in her to get back on her grind. She began to get back into the swing of a consistent regimen. She says,

"To answer the question, why do I work out? It's because I just cannot live the lifestyle of not doing so."

It's also important to her because it makes her look and feel good by staying consistent. In January of 2010 she became the Assistant Track & Field Coach at Rutgers - Newark. She's passionate about her job and it's from this passion that she continues to work out to lead by example. Practicing what she preaches to her athletes.

There were times in her career where Janine was derailed by some injuries, and she wasn't able to compete. She struggled with this because she didn't know what to do to get better fast. It seemed like nothing her athletic trainers were doing or suggesting for her was working. It almost drove her to just quit and give up…but she didn't. She did some research on her own and it helped. She also struggled with not knowing what to do once she began, because it was always given to her.

"I was so used to being given a workout on the track or in the weight room and following through with it because I knew that the person initiating the workout had to know what they were talking about."

She also says,

"Not working out because I didn't know what to do was an excuse, and I could no longer allow myself to think that doing a little exercise here and there was good enough."

It was a struggle but she did what she had to do to get to where she wanted to be. With her determination to find out information and not be hindered from this excuse any longer, she learned to create workouts for herself and her student-athletes.

She discovered what worked for her and you can too if you believe in yourself. She says, *"a wise man once told me, good enough never is!"* Janine believes this is a great motivational message that can be applied to life in general. Knowing that you can always be better will help you achieve the unthinkable. Don't be afraid to ask for help, there is nothing wrong with not knowing but there is something wrong with ignoring the fact that you don't know.

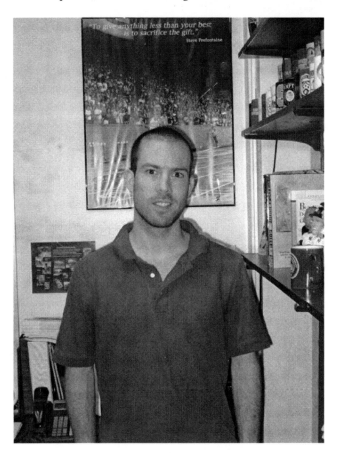

This next gentleman always finds a way to get an answer when he doesn't have one. He knows the importance of his goals, so challenges are nothing more than a speed bump in the road. Slows him down but doesn't stop him.

William Seaman, high school counselor and track coach. Exercising comes natural to him because he has been doing it for a large part of his life. Here's why he exercises,

> *"I began running in high school, and I have been running ever since. At different points I have trained for different reasons. In high school I competed on the Cross-Country, Indoor, and Outdoor teams. After that, I raced mostly 5k's in my 20's, and I trained mostly for distance, without the incentive of an organized track team. I did not race that often, but I would work out hard and push myself because I liked the feeling of being in great shape. I have run two marathons, which are*

tough because I really don't run enough mileage to train to race them fast, but they were a tremendous experience."

This took a lot of dedication on his part. Even though everything he did was part of track and field, different training methods were required for it. He didn't know going into each different area what to do, but he knew he wanted to be successful so he found out to make it happen. William found ways to make it part of his lifestyle,

"Although I still enjoy the basic fitness aspect of running, this has allowed me to bring the competitive aspect back to my training. It also allows me to be in shape to run with the athletes that I coach from time to time."

Lack of knowledge shouldn't stop you from achieving your goals. It can, in a way, be a motivator to also expand your knowledge. That's exactly what he did. He found the answers to his questions which taught him something new, as well as helped him become a better athlete and coach. William came to a point in his life where he didn't know what to do. He ran injury free for majority of his life but then tragedy struck and he was faced with a semi-serious injury. He developed IT Band Syndrome (Ileotibial Band), which is a tendon-like muscle that extends from the gluteus medias to the side of the knee. The inflammation and soreness occurs in the knee, as the tightness in the IT Band causes it to rub against bones in the knee area. He says,

" I was running injury free for mostly my entire life, this was a difficult obstacle to face since it greatly limited my running for about three years, and sometimes prevented me from running at all. What held me back was the lack of knowledge of how to improve my condition. This required much more than the knowledge that I had, and I feared that the situation would never improve. I feared that my days of running hard were over. This fear caused me to hold back from learning more about my injury. I would wait until my knee did not hurt and then I would resume my workouts, but the knee would always become inflamed again, which caused me to stop running again."

Instead of letting it haunt him for the rest of his life, he did something.

"There were times when I considered giving in to my IT Band Syndrome and putting my running career behind me, even though this is something that I did not want to do. But I did not want an injury to

be the reason that I stopped running. I realized that I had to learn about the condition, which meant that I had to learn about more about the mechanics and physiology of running. This required determination, but it also asked for a sense of patience. My condition could not be fixed with a snap of the fingers and it would take time to see the effects of the physical therapy and conditioning that I needed to do."

When asked about tips for other people who may have faced this excuse he said,

"Lack of knowledge can result in the fear of the unknown. You can battle this by realizing that the only way you can improve your situation is to face reality."

Once he overcame this, he was ready to make the change and he did.

"Rather than avoiding a fearful situation, it is best to go right at it and to face it head on. Embrace your fear and anxiety. Then look at the facts of the situation and decide what you need to learn. As a beginner, get help from someone who knows about the type of physical activity that you are trying to pursue. If you are experience already, but want to get to the next level, be willing to take in new knowledge to incorporate into what you already know."

If you allow yourself to only rely on past knowledge it can lead to dead ends and repeated mistakes, which can only lead to frustration and disappointment. In the end it will only enable you to fall victim to this excuse.

"Taking the shortcut in life only creates temporary gratification. A gratification which will only turn to regret because it will set you back further than you were when you began. Do it right it stays for life."

2 THE RESULTS AREN'T COMING FAST ENOUGH

f the perfect body came in a pill, everyone would have one already. Since something like this doesn't exist; you're going to have to put in the work to get what you want. Quick fixes don't last long anyway. They only put you in a position to become worse off than when you began the process. If you've been looking for a quick route to fitness, consider the way you take care of your car. Your car has an issue, so you take it to get fixed. The mechanic says your problem takes 10 hours to fix it, but there's a quicker two-hour way to *temporarily* fix the problem. Would you want them to take the quicker way to fix your car or the 10 hour way which will correct the problem for good? No one would pick the "quick fix" for their car because they know that it could ultimately lead to even bigger problems from when they first went to the mechanic to get their car fixed. So, if you wouldn't do it for your car which can be replaced; why would you do it for your life when you only get one?

It seems as if individuals no longer want to or enjoy working hard to achieve their goals. If things came to you so easily, don't you think at some point you'd get bored? The thing is, if people didn't wait so long to get started on the path to improved health and wellness, it actually wouldn't be as hard or even take as long. More often than not, people start looking for a "quick fix" after they've brushed off their need to get in shape. You had time, it just wasn't that important to you. Now, you've revisited your "New Year's resolution" and you want to get in shape; maybe for the summer, a trip, wedding, or just because you need to improve your health; because now it's a *priority*…sort of. The unfortunate part to your moment of realization is that you've waited so long, the time to accomplish it seems shorten. Hence the need for the quick fix. Here's the biggest obstacle with "quick fixes", they come with complications…complications which can affect your health and your physical appearance in the long run. All a quick fix does is patch up a surface issue; it doesn't address the real problem.

A quick fix can be a binge diet, not eating, or even over exercising. None of these things are maintainable for a long period of time and are just unhealthy for your normal body function. Since this isn't a sustainable mode of weight loss, eventually you will revert back to your old habits. Many times it will lead you right back to the place you were originally or worse. So what purpose did that quick fix actually serve? Nothing! What you're supposed to do is take the time to get to the place you want. By doing this, you go through the process of understanding the steps behind weight loss and being healthy, which will also allow you to maintain the results of your hard work. Start off slow and improve in small steps, remember it's a process. It's an attainable goal; you just have to have patience and remain positive. Before you know it, you will be where you want to be.

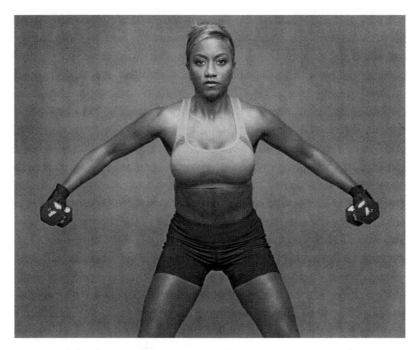

To qualify this further, Dr. Joy Ohayia is a woman who is in the health and wellness industry. She doesn't have to work out but makes it her business to do so. Below is her story.

Dr. Joy Ohayia, is the author of *Don't Let "IT" Get You! An Empowering Health and Fitness Guide for Women* and *Blueprint for Success – Proven Strategies for Success and Survival*. She is also a motivational speaker, Total Wellness Expert, a mother of two and is 47 years young. Dr. Joy is passionate about motivating people in all areas of life. She accomplishes this through a fully comprehensive program that she provides for private, corporate, and virtual clients; enabling them to achieve and maintain their wellness goals. More information about her services can be found at her website, www.drxjoy.com.

Although she works in the health and wellness industry, that's not what makes her work out. Prior to embarking on her journey in the wellness field, she had a 20 year executive level career in corporate America. Despite working in corporate America she managed to keep herself physically and mentally fit. When asked why she works out she said,

"Exercise is called the most potent antidote!! My daily work out regime is an integral part of my lifestyle as it has a multi-faceted purpose: first it jump starts my metabolism as workout routines are completed

in the early morning; second: it helps reduce stress; third, a sense of accomplishment is achieved before the other part of my day begins. All of us have "competing priorities" that take up our time; the motivating message received by my clients I follow as well – take care of yourself first and you will be in a better position to take care of everyone else – It is NEVER too late to begin your journey to achieving total wellness!"

Dr. Joy continues her exercise regimen because she wants to maintain her healthy lifestyle. She understands that patience is a virtue and great things come to those who wait. So when she sets goals, she plans them out knowing that it won't happen overnight. She says,

"You cannot achieve physical wellness naturally by taking one pill that will do the trick. Consistency is the key and results will prevail."

She realizes that to achieve total wellness it's a journey and as with any journey, it takes time to get to the end.

Helping others is her passion. So when I asked her what she could suggest to others who may fall victim to this "excuse illness" she answered,

"Before setting health and wellness goals, determine what behaviors you are TRULY ready to change. If you think you are doing fine and don't need to work on WELLNESS, get REAL with yourself! We all have behaviors we can work on and improve in this area. WRITE DOWN what your ideal health picture should look like. When in your life did you feel and look your VERY best?"

Dr. Joy has developed six specific steps of how you can achieve your goals, while understanding the process and that it will take time to get there. Her six steps include:

1. **Create a vision statement based on how you will look, feel and behave.** Here is a sample wellness vision: "I will become a more balanced, less stressed, even tempered person and will make health my top priority."

2. **Set three month goals based on your vision statement.** Six month and one year goals can also be set; however, setting three month goals gives urgency to start working toward the goal today. It's also best to only work on three to five changes at a time. When we try to make too many changes at once we can feel overwhelmed and defeated.

3. **Determine your INTERNAL MOTIVATORS for**

change and put them in writing. Why do you want to "run a marathon", "lose 20 pounds", "start a weight-training program", etc.?

4. **Determine your obstacles, I call them "IT's".** "IT's" are competing priorities that hinder us from achieving the things we want in life. Do your best friends disapprove of your healthy eating? Are you a night owl, but have a goal to start running early in the mornings? List all the people or habits that are keeping you from achieving your goals and come up with a strategy as to how you are going to get around those obstacles.

5. **What 3 things can you do this week to work toward your 3-month goals?** Make certain you are at least 80% sure you can achieve your weekly goals. If you are not at least 80% certain, you need to cut back on the goal. Maybe run only two mornings this week instead of the four you thought you could do.

6. **To whom will you be accountable?** Many of us need a hand or a shoulder on which to lean. Solicit support from one or two family members or a close friend that will positively support your efforts through your journey of achieving optimum health.

It is her belief that if you follow these six steps you will have the ability to reach any goal you may have.

Patience is truly a virtue. Knowing this will not only help you out in the world of exercise, but also with keeping yourself healthy and in life. Here is a gentleman who knows all too well that hard work pays off in the end.

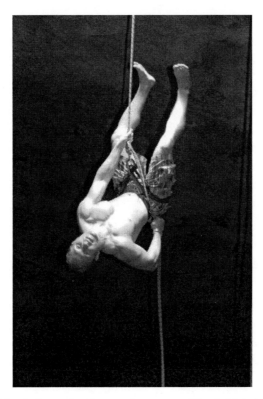

Gregory Hoak, Jr. is the fitness director at Hatfield Athletic Club. He is also a strength coach, personal trainer, and fitness consultant. He works out for a few different reasons.

> *"I started exercising at an early age and I always have found it to be a vital component of leading a high functioning lifestyle. My daily routine is very demanding and at times stressful, and I use exercise to help keep my mind and body ready to meet these demands."*

Demands can come from any source; it can be your family, job, or even your social life. As Greg says, these demands can become stressful. Exercise is something that can help combat these stressors. Additionally Greg states,

> *"I find that exercise has helped improve my stamina, strength, and has a major impact in helping me maintain a positive attitude to tackle any obstacles that I need to overcome."*

It's all about staying positive, knowing that in the end all of your efforts will not be in vain. Despite his profession he would still work out...

"Yes. I exercised as a student, manual laborer, and now exercise professionally. I feel that daily exercise is vital even for the individual that has an extremely active job. In most professions, repetitive movements are common and it is vital that individuals perform strength training exercise and active and passive stretching in order to help correct certain muscle imbalances that can lead to occupational overuse injuries. Individuals with less active occupations, where there are long periods of sitting, should also consider emphasizing the cardiovascular component of exercise. Overall, it is best to balance your exercise routine by including strength training, flexibility, and cardiovascular (aerobic) exercise."

Everyone has heard the saying "hard work will pay off", but when your results aren't coming as fast as you want, it may be hard to believe. It can be discouraging but you have to find your motivation – your special reason for wanting to exercise. That will keep you focused. Greg's focus is here...

"As a student of exercise science, I know that the body changes by making small yet sustainable adaptations to the applied stresses of exercise. Because I have made exercise a part of my everyday routine, I have noticed small improvements over the last 15 years that have added up to creating a strong mind and healthy body."

People often overlook the mental benefits of exercise. Seeing yourself succeed in your exercise program can make you more willing to push yourself through other things in life.

"I have never judged myself on appearance or short term gain, and I never use the scale, stop watch, or tape measure as a tool to set goals for myself. My overall goal throughout has been to feel proud of my efforts day in and day out. Due to this outlook, I can truly say that I am proud of myself."

This is a great way to look at your efforts. You are more than your appearance, and you should be proud of all your progress no matter how small.

"Perception is the key to breaking through any of life's road blocks. Start changing your perception of exercise by the way you set your goals. Losing 10 pounds seems to be a good goal but where do you go from there?"

How you view exercise is also important (perception). This determines how focused you will be in achieving your weight loss goals. Another tip he suggests is,

> "…having a better starting point would be to set a goal of exercising for 30 minutes every day. This can be easily measured and helps fill the role of a short and long term goal. The first bench mark you hit may be losing the first 10 pounds of body fat or gaining the first 10 pounds of muscle. After you have this routine set it will become easier to set these benchmarks, choose a method of exercise to get there, and bust through those road blocks."

These are just examples. Try them. If they work, great! If not, don't worry; a solution is definitely out there. The question is; are you willing to put *in* the work to find *what* works?

"Time is relative, based on what you deem as being important. There is a need to create a balance in order to accomplish the things you want in your life. Time is not the factor. You are!!!"

I DON'T HAVE ENOUGH TIME

This is the number one excuse that people come up with to not work out. "I don't have enough time." A person will argue with all their strength to convince you that the things that they do on a daily basis keep them from being able to work out. "I have to go to work, I have school, I have to clean, and take care of the baby." The list can go on forever. I always find it funny that these same people who claim to not have time to live a healthier lifestyle will miraculously find the time for other things they want to accomplish. The sad thing is that they can't see it's only an excuse that they have created for themselves. I have had this discussion more times than I can recall. I have even shown people ways they can create the time but, in many cases, they have chosen not to because other things are more important to them than working out.

Why aren't you making the time? Could it be because you're afraid of not reaching your goals that you would set out to accomplish? Could you be scheduling your day to avoid doing things that you find difficult? Is it that you really don't have the desire to work out and commit to the process of working out like you may think you do? Saying that you don't have time is only an excuse for avoiding something that you don't want to. The relevance of things in one's life is how you equate the balance of time. Until you can sit back and tell yourself that this particular thing such as *working out* is important to you, and that you're going to make sure you incorporate it in your day, you will "never have time." You have time to watch your favorite show(s), or to go hang out with your friends, don't you? But, at the same time, you don't have time to work out. It's because in your mind those things are more important than your desire to get healthy. Not to say that you can't do those things, but how about hanging out with friends while doing some exercise, or during the commercials of your favorite show(s) you could do pushups and sit ups. Every little bit counts towards the ultimate goal which should not only be to look good, but more importantly to feel great and live a healthy lifestyle. That's the real victory - to always remain healthy. A nice physique does not equate to a healthy body.

I'm sure we all have heard many different reasons (excuses) as to why an individual does not have the time to work out. They always have this or that to do. Then after they do this and that, there is still is more to do. Blah blah blah, it's a never ending saga of excuses. But the woman I'm about to introduce is the epitome of a goal achiever. She is someone who refuses to make excuses or allow obstacles to stop her plans. Pay close attention to what she has to say.

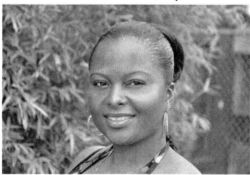

Tamara Hawkins – prenatal educator and lactation consultant from 9am-5pm, business owner managing her own company Stork and Cradle, certified Holistic Health Counselor and a single mother of a teenage daughter.

Tamara works out for a few reasons….

"I work out because I want to look good. Come on let's be honest. It's the day and age of SEXY. I have to work out because heart disease

is the number one killer of women and diabetes is 2-4 times higher in African American and Hispanic woman than our Caucasian sisters."

This is just the beginning of her motivation. Despite all she does in the day, she makes it her business to get her work outs in. She even wakes up at 5am so she can work out and then get her day started.

"I exercise because I need to be a healthy role model for my teenage daughter. I have a desire to live to be a strong beautiful senior woman like those featured in the Essence magazine feature 'Fabulous over Fifty'."

Her key is, having more than one reason to drive and motivate her. She understands that it's not only about looking good, but also realizing the other benefits of working out as well. Tamara says,

"Working out is one of the things I do to care for myself. I feel good, I'm energized, and I'm pumped after a workout. Yes, it hurts. Yes, it burns but in the end it feels good and it's worth it."

With her lifestyle, Tamara could choose to use many of the different "reasons" not to exercise, but she doesn't. One reason for not letting this excuse hold her back is because,

"Time waits for no one and when I know I'm getting lazy I just give myself that look in the mirror like, Girl, you better get your act together and I make it my priority to workout. I drag myself out of bed in the morning and go to the gym after work because I know it's going to make a difference on my self esteem, my stamina, and my health."

She knows what is important. For her, it's her health, being there for her daughter, other family and her clients. If she isn't healthy then she can't do those things. Tamara also says,

"I schedule my workouts just like I schedule my clients. Oh, and watching the Biggest Loser is a great motivator! Just watching them push themselves gets me excited and lets me know I can do anything."

Hard work will pay off you, just have to get motivated and stay focused. Making time is a something that's hard to do. Tamara continues on saying,

"What I found is that it's not all about working out. In order to be able to get up at 5:30am to exercise I have to watch what I eat and

make sure I'm not eating heaving foods the day prior. It really slows me down and makes me sluggish in the morning."

She pays attention to what her body is telling her and listens so she can be successful in reaching her goals.

Tamara knows what works best for her, and if that doesn't work anymore she finds another solution. All problems have a solution. You just have to be willing to go through the process of finding it. Here's a tip she has for single mothers who think they don't have time,

> *"...first for all the mothers, if your child is over the age of five they can help you around the house and save you some time to exercise. Teach them to clean their room, put away their toys, books, shoes etc. Teach them to pull out clothes to wear for school and sort clothes for the laundry. Don't try to do it all yourself."*

You can also create a schedule for yourself. Write down everything you do each day making sure it's the important and essential things, and exactly how many hours it takes up. You will be surprised where you could fit things in. Even if it's only ten minutes at a time, every little bit helps. For others she says,

> *"...make your work outs your priority. I received a few huffs and puffs and remarks when I declined nights out with friends but I needed to wake up and exercise. My evenings can be unpredictable while running a corporation so I make sure I get in my exercise in the morning. But do make time for play and I have fun!"*

It's all about prioritizing what's important to you. Once you make your life, health and well-being a priority in your life, you will see how easy it becomes to make the time. People often tend to forget themselves and get lost in the shuffle.

Still not convinced? You don't just have to take my word for it. Here's another person who has limited time but still finds the time to exercise. Why, because it is something that he actually wants to do.

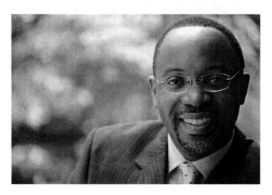

Andrew Morrison, president of Small Business Camp, trainer and International business coach. He inspires people through his motivational speaking and teaches them how to turn their concepts into cash with less time and effort.

Andrew chooses to get his exercise by practicing martial arts and he also makes time to jog. Soon he plans to train and participate in a marathon. When asks why he chooses to work out he replied,

> *"I started out by running track in high school and then went on to run track in college. I discovered that my best years academically in college were also the years I was running track." He then states, "As I have gotten older I have found the connection with exercise and the ability to process information and the ability to deal with stress."*

Andrew feels that exercise isn't something that people should view as something added to their daily lives and activities, but as something critical to help them think more effectively with the ability to deal with stressful situations.

Despite heading a multi-million dollar company and traveling all over the world, Andrew still manages to create the time to get some exercise in. He says,

> *"I understand the health benefits and the mental benefits of exercise. So I am compelled to exercise."*

Andrew feels the number one reason why people don't reach their goals is because they weren't serious about reaching their goals. He believes people aren't serious about it because they really didn't understand the benefits that come along with exercise. He says,

> *"People often do more to avoid pain then they will to gain pleasure. I know how painful it is for me not to make money. I make my money*

based upon the quality of my thoughts, and exercise provides me with more powerful and more compelling thoughts."

His driving force to always make time to exercise is his fear of not being able to make money. The best way to conqueror your fear is to allow it to be a driving force to help you achieve your goals. Many of the fears you may have about exercise could be turned into a motivating factor. People do it all the time, but it is up to you to make the switch.

If you want to achieve your goals you first have to find what works best for you. Andrew uses a quote by George Fraser which states, "*it takes teamwork to make the dream work.*" He also suggests,

"The best thing that you could to is to find a buddy, find a buddy, and find a buddy. Do not make the commitment to exercising all by yourself. Find someone who is willing to support you in ensuring the success of your goals."

You can join a walking group or club. When you begin to work within a team, when you're down someone else will pull you up and vice versa. He says,

"Before you begin your planning your exercise goals have the new attitude of finding a workout buddy. Or if you can't find a workout buddy hire a trainer that's also a good route."

It is possible to reach your goals on your own, but it is a harder task to accomplish, and in order to get there you will have to be strong and stay positive.

There you have it; the top 10 most used excuses to avoid exercise. Sure there are plenty more but you and I both know that the ones listed in this book are ones you use most. Am I here to bash you about it, no. Am I here to beat you over the head about the importance of exercise? Sounds ideal, but not at all. The purpose of this book is to uncover these "excuses", offer you solutions to the problem, and share with you others who have experienced similar situations, as well as moved passed the roadblock. At the end of the day, that's all it truly is…a roadblock.

Challenges are what they are, challenges. If we didn't have them, how would we know how strong our faith is, the test of our endurance and the gumption within our heart? Exercising and maintaining a healthy lifestyle is a challenge. We all go through the same thing, the difference is our will to stay on course and get to the other side. You've heard the saying "what's good for the goose, isn't good for the gander", and I agree. Not everything suggestion will be the savior to your problems, but it's a start and that's what you need…a start.

As noted in Chapter 6 [and found in the Appendix], use the self-assessment test to gage your readiness in beginning your workout regimen. Don't be afraid to write down your goals and be real with yourself. Being realistic will help in overcoming the excuses. Let's be clear, there's nothing wrong with having ambitious goals, in order to determine how strong we are, we must move out of our comfort zone [relative to Chapter 9]; however, when setting the bar too high upon starting something new or simply reactivating a lifestyle that has been on pause; you risk the chance of disappointment. This is what you want to avoid. Start small and gradually increase the deliverables that you'd like to achieve. When you see progression in your goals, it's encouraging and ensures you're on the right track. Be realistic but don't doubt your strength. It's a balancing act.

Remember the S.M.A.R.T. discussed in Chapter 5? Without clearly setting S.M.A.R.T. goals, it will increase the level of challenge with working to achieve your goals. There is no need to make it harder than it needs to be, *think, plan, execute.* Organize your thoughts, develop your strategy, get your plan down on paper and implement. Set reminders and follow-ups to ensure you stay on track. Knowledge is power, discover what tools are necessary to enhance and develop your workout regimen and healthier eating habits. Refer back to Chapter 9; there are plenty of websites, magazines and other informational tools available to educate yourself on the best modes of achieving your goals. You just have to place it in your mind to do it and be liberated by the thought of increasing your knowledge on health and wellness. Furthermore, you can use this knowledge to assist others who share the same struggles. Sharing what you've learned is also a great motivational tool. By encouraging others, you become encouraged yourself in wanting to help other achieve their goals, much like you.

Does creating a routine sound familiar [refer back to Chapter 8]? Of course it does, that's what it is important to train your mind to believe that nothing or no one can stand in the way of achieving your goals. As mentioned in the book, you are your biggest motivator. If you can't encourage yourself, then who can? By adding structure to your lifestyle change, it gives you something to look forward to each day. Don't forget to add some variety to your workout such as taking classes and various forms of instructional aerobics [discussed in Chapter 8]. The mind is a powerful thing and without it, things can get rough. Having the ability to train your mind to focus on the positives in your life and not the negatives; helps to re-focus your purpose and see them through. Once you take ownership of the process, training your mind will begin to reshape your thinking towards a better you and achieving your goals.

The only "thing" that is preventing you from success is YOU! Remember, you can focus on the thought that possibilities are endless. The time is not to begin to define a new you but to begin today with a clear mind, new attitude and support system that keeps you focused and upbeat. Get started today and you're life will NEVER be the same.

"Reshape Your Body & Your Mind"

QUOTES AND REFLECTIONS

This section was created to enable you to carefully re-read and reflect on the 10 quotes found in this book. After you re-read them, write down what about the quote you find helpful. Think about how it relates to where you are in life, and where you would like to be. You could also write down a situation that each quote relates to in your life. The blank pages after the quotes were created to give you space to create and develop your own words of inspiration. These words that you use to push yourself toward your goals may one day become quotes that inspire others to reach for their own greatness. The time is now, grasp every second of it!!!

"If you push yourself beyond your perceived limits nothing will ever be unattainable."

Reggie Lamptey

_____

_____

_____

_____

_____

_____

_____

_____

_____

"Once you have begun to trickle into the realm of being comfortable you have given up and settled for your present state."

Reggie Lamptey

_____
_____
_____
_____
_____
_____
_____
_____
_____

"Creating your own excitement will lead to powerful results."

Reggie Lamptey

_____
_____
_____
_____
_____
_____
_____
_____
_____

"Going the extra mile and doing some extra can go a long way to endless possibilities. Anything less would limit your true potential."

Reggie Lamptey

_____

_____

_____

_____

_____

_____

_____

_____

_____

"The ability to find happiness and greatness within you can avoid the demise of compliments in the form of distractions."

Reggie Lamptey

_____

_____

_____

_____

_____

_____

_____

_____

_____

"Finding the connection of importance to one's self is the key to success, focus and continued motivation in life."

Reggie Lamptey

_____

_____

_____

_____

_____

_____

_____

_____

_____

"Simple sacrifice must be made in order for the true vision to be accomplished."

Reggie Lamptey

_____

_____

_____

_____

_____

_____

_____

_____

_____

"Just because you don't have the answer right in front of you, doesn't mean it can't be found."

Reggie Lamptey

"Taking the shortcut in life only creates temporary gratification. A gratification which will only turn to regret because it will set you back further than you were when you began. Do it right it stays for life."

Reggie Lamptey

"Time is relative, based on what you deem as being important. There is a need to create a balance in order to accomplish the things you want in your life. Time is not the factor. You are!!!"

Reggie Lamptey

_____

_____

_____

_____

_____

_____

_____

_____

_____

_____

CPSIA information can be obtained at www.ICGtesting.com
Printed in the USA
LVOW072220141211

259491LV00003B/123/P